Mind Diet
Cookbook
for Seniors Over 60

Over 80
Recipes to
Keep your Brain Healthy and
Avoid Cognitive Deterioration

Dr. Olivia Tastewell

© 2024 by Dr Olivia Tastewell

The recipes and information in this book are based on the author's personal experience and research. They are not intended to replace the advice of your doctor or health care provider. Please consult your doctor before making any changes to your diet or lifestyle. The author and publisher are not responsible for any adverse effects or consequences resulting from the use of any of the recipes or information in this book.

The author hopes that this book will inspire you to enjoy cooking and eating healthy and delicious food. She welcomes your feedback and suggestions and invites you to share your recipes and stories with her. Thank you for choosing this book and supporting the author's work.

Dr Olivia Tastewell
Author of Crock Pot Cookbook for College Students
Email: droliviatastewell@gmail.com

TABLE OF CONTENT

INTRODUCTION

WHEN PEOPLE GET OLDER, THEY MAY experience a variety of obstacles to their health and well-being. One of the most crucial elements of aging is keeping your brain healthy and avoiding cognitive deterioration. Cognitive decline is the slow loss of memory, thinking, and reasoning skills, which can affect one's capacity to do everyday tasks and enjoy life. Some of the common concerns addressed by seniors over 60 regarding cognitive impairment are:

- **Alzheimer's:** This disease and other types of dementia are progressive brain illnesses that cause irreparable damage to brain cells and impair cognitive ability. According to the World Health Organization, dementia affects around 50 million people globally, with that figure anticipated to increase to 152 million by 2050. Alzheimer's disease is the leading cause of dementia, accounting for 60% to 70% of cases.

- **Mild cognitive impairment (MCI):** is a condition characterized by a minor but perceptible deterioration in cognitive abilities such as memory and language. MCI does not impair daily functioning, but it raises the chance of acquiring dementia. MCI affects around 15-20% of adults over the age of 65.

- **Depression and anxiety:** These are typical mental health issues that can affect anybody, but they are more common among the elderly. Depression and anxiety can impair one's mood, energy, sleep, appetite, and attention. They can also accelerate cognitive deterioration and raise the risk of dementia. Depression is the most frequent mental or neurological condition, affecting around 20% of persons over the age of 60.

- **Stroke and vascular dementia:** These are disorders caused by decreased blood supply to the brain, which can cause brain damage and impair cognitive function. A stroke is a medical emergency that happens when a blood artery in the brain breaks or becomes blocked by a clot. Vascular dementia is a kind of dementia that develops following a stroke or series of strokes. Stroke is the second-largest cause of mortality and the third-greatest cause of disability globally. Vascular dementia affects around 3% of adults aged 65 and older.

- **Nutritional deficiencies and chronic illnesses:** These can have an impact on both general health and well-being, as well as brain health. Nutritional deficiencies, such as low vitamin B12, folate, iron, and zinc levels, can result in anemia, weariness, weakness, and cognitive impairment. Chronic disorders including diabetes, hypertension, heart disease, and obesity can lead to increased inflammation, oxidative stress, and vascular damage, all of which can affect brain cells and cognitive functioning.

Fortunately, there are methods for preventing or delaying cognitive decline and enhancing brain health. One of the most successful and fun methods is to have a healthy and balanced diet that nourishes and protects the brain from harm. This is where the MIND Diet comes in. The MIND diet is an acronym for Mediterranean-DASH Intervention for Neurodegenerative Delay. It combines two well-known diets that have been shown to improve cardiovascular health and prevent chronic diseases: the Mediterranean diet and the DASH (Dietary Approaches to Stop Hypertension) diet. The MIND diet emphasizes foods that have been demonstrated to improve brain function and prevent dementia, such as green leafy vegetables, berries, nuts, olive oil, salmon, and whole grains. It also restricts items that can affect the brain, such as red meat, butter, cheese, sweets, and fried meals.

The MIND diet benefits not only your brain but also your body and taste sensibilities. It's simple to follow, versatile, and tasty. It can aid with weight loss, lower blood pressure, and cholesterol levels, and lessen your risk of diabetes and heart disease. It can also improve your attitude, energy level, and mental clarity. And, most crucially, it can help you maintain your memory and cognitive abilities as you age.

This cookbook is your complete guide to following the MIND diet and reaping its advantages.

It includes over 70 dishes that are simple, fast, and delicious. They are appropriate for persons at all levels who are following the MIND diet or wish to try it. Whether you're searching for breakfast, lunch, supper, snacks, or dessert ideas, you'll find something to satisfy your hunger and fuel your brain. Each dish also contains nutritional information and suggestions for how to customize it to your interests and requirements.

So what are you waiting for? Grab your apron and cookbook, and prepare to embark on a culinary journey that will benefit your mind and life. Bon appétit!

Chapter One

Overview of the MIND Diet

I know you must have probably heard of the phrase "You are what you eat". This is particularly true in terms of brain health. What you eat has a significant influence on your memory, cognition, emotions, and general well-being. That is why eating the correct meals for your brain is one of the most effective ways to prevent or slow cognitive decline and dementia. But what nutrients are best for the brain? How do you include them in your everyday diet? This is where the MIND diet steps in. The MIND diet is a scientifically established eating plan that can help you nourish and preserve your brain. In this chapter, we will discuss the MIND diet and its key components. We will also go over the benefits and drawbacks of following the MIND diet, as well as some advice on how to get started and keep to it.

Main foods and food groups

The acronym MIND refers to Mediterranean-DASH Intervention for Neurodegenerative Delay. It combines the Mediterranean diet with the DASH diet, both of which have been shown to improve cardiovascular health and avoid chronic illnesses.

Green leafy vegetables, berries, almonds, olive oil, salmon, and whole grains are among the items on the MIND diet that have been proven to promote brain function and help prevent dementia. It also restricts items that can be harmful to the brain, including red meat, butter, cheese, sweets, and fried meals.

The MIND diet is made up of 15 food types, 10 of which are brain-healthy and 5 of which are brain-harmful. The ten brain-healthy dietary categories include:

- **Green leafy vegetables:** These are high in antioxidants, vitamins, minerals, and fiber, which can help protect the brain from oxidation and inflammation. They also include folate, which is required for DNA synthesis and repair. Green leafy vegetables consist of spinach, kale, collard greens, Swiss chard, and lettuce. You should strive to consume at least one serving of green leafy vegetables each day and six servings per week.
- **Other vegetables:** These are high in antioxidants, vitamins, minerals, and fiber, which can aid the brain. They also include phytochemicals including carotenoids, flavonoids, and glucosinolates, which can influence cellular signaling and gene expression. Broccoli, cauliflower, carrots, tomatoes, peppers,

and squash are among more vegetable options. You should consume at least one serving of other veggies each day, and at least five servings per week.

- **Berries:** are high in antioxidants, particularly anthocyanins, which help protect the brain from oxidative stress and inflammation. They also contain anti-amyloid and anti-tau properties, preventing the buildup of harmful proteins linked to Alzheimer's disease. Blueberries, strawberries, raspberries, blackberries, and cranberries are all berries. You should consume at least two servings of berries every week.

- **Nuts:** These are high in healthy fats, particularly omega-3 fatty acids, which help increase blood flow and decrease inflammation in the brain. They also include protein, fiber, vitamins E, magnesium, and selenium, all of which can help with brain function and structure. Walnuts, almonds, pistachios, cashews, and pecans are all varieties of nuts. You should strive to consume at least one serving of nuts each day and at least five servings per week.

- **Olive oil:** The MIND diet's major fat source is olive oil. It has a lot of monounsaturated fatty acids, which can help decrease cholesterol and blood pressure while also preventing atherosclerosis.

It also includes polyphenols, which can help protect the brain from oxidative stress and inflammation. Use olive oil as your main cooking oil and sprinkle it over salads and vegetables. You should eat at least three tablespoons of olive oil every day.

- **Fish:** This is a high-protein food that contains omega-3 fatty acids, particularly DHA and EPA, which help improve brain function and structure. Omega-3 fatty acids can also influence gene expression, neuronal plasticity, and neurogenesis. Salmon, tuna, sardines, mackerel, and herring are all fish. You should consume at least one dish of fish every week.

- **Whole grains:** These contain complex carbs, fiber, and B vitamins, which can offer energy and sustenance to the brain. They can also aid with blood sugar and insulin regulation, as well as metabolic syndrome prevention. Whole grains comprise brown rice, oats, quinoa, barley, and bulgur. You should strive to consume at least three servings of whole grains each day.

- **Poultry:** Poultry is an excellent source of protein and B vitamins, particularly vitamin B12, which can help with brain function and structure. Vitamin B12 is necessary for the production of neurotransmitters, myelin, and DNA. Poultry includes chickens, turkeys, and ducks.

You should strive to consume at least two servings of poultry per week.

- **Beans:** Rich in protein, fiber, iron, and folate, which can aid the brain. They can also assist in decreasing cholesterol and blood pressure, as well as prevent diabetes. Beans consist of black beans, kidney beans, chickpeas, lentils, and soybeans. You should strive to consume at least three servings of beans weekly.

- **Wine:** This contains a modest amount of alcohol, which can have a protective impact on the brain when drunk in moderation. Alcohol can improve blood flow and decrease inflammation in the brain. It can also increase the release of acetylcholine, a neurotransmitter important in memory and learning. Wine, particularly red wine, contains resveratrol, a polyphenol that can protect the brain against oxidative stress and inflammation. You should try to consume no more than one glass of wine every day.

The five dietary categories that can affect the brain are:

- **Red meat:** is heavy in saturated fat and cholesterol, which can raise the risk of heart disease and stroke. It also includes iron, which can lead to oxidative stress and inflammation in the brain.

Red meat consists of beef, hog, lamb, and veal. You should try to consume no more than three portions of red meat each week, ideally fewer.

- **Butter and margarine:** are heavy in saturated and trans fats, which can elevate cholesterol and blood pressure while also damaging brain blood vessels. They also contain palmitic acid, which can disrupt insulin signaling and glucose metabolism in the brain. You should consume no more than one tablespoon of butter or margarine every day, ideally less.

- **Cheese:** Cheese is heavy in saturated fat and salt, which can raise the risk of heart disease and stroke. It also includes casein, which may cause inflammation and oxidative stress in the brain. You should try to consume no more than one serving of cheese each week, ideally less.

- **Pastries and sweets**: These are heavy in refined carbs and added sugars, which can raise blood sugar and insulin levels, leading to metabolic syndrome. They also include advanced glycation end products (AGEs), which have the potential to harm brain proteins and cells. Pastries and sweets include cakes, pies, cookies, doughnuts, candies, and ice cream. You should strive to consume no more than four servings of pastries and sweets each week, ideally fewer.

- **Fried and fast foods:** are high in saturated fat, trans fat, salt, and calories, raising the risk of obesity, diabetes, hypertension, and heart disease. They also include acrylamide, which can cause neurotoxicity and inflammation. Fried and quick food items include french fries, hamburgers, pizza, nuggets, and hot dogs. You should limit your intake of fried and fast foods to one serving per week, ideally fewer.

Advantages and Challenges

The MIND diet has several advantages over other diets, including:

- It is supported by strong scientific data and clinical trials that demonstrate its effectiveness in avoiding cognitive decline and dementia. Morris et al. (2015) found that the MIND diet can reduce the risk of Alzheimer's disease by up to 53%, with moderate adherence lowering the risk by up to 35%.
- It is simple to follow and adaptable since it does not need stringent calorie tracking, portion restriction, or food elimination. It also allows for occasional pleasures such as wine, cheese, and sweets, provided they are enjoyed in moderation and within the suggested limits.

-

- It is tasty and gratifying since it offers a wide range of dishes and flavors to suit diverse tastes and preferences. It also contains meals high in protein, fiber, and healthy fats, which can help you stay full and energetic for longer.
- It benefits not only your brain but also your body and entire wellness. It can aid with weight loss, lower blood pressure, and cholesterol levels, and lessen your risk of diabetes and heart disease. It can also improve your attitude, energy level, and mental clarity.

However, the MIND diet has some disadvantages, such as:

- Some of the items indicated on the MIND diet may be difficult to locate or buy, particularly if you live in a location where fresh vegetables, seafood, nuts, and olive oil are in short supply or costly. You may need to hunt for other sources or alternatives for some of the items advised by the MIND diet, such as:

- **Frozen or canned vegetables and fruits:** These are less expensive and more convenient than fresh ones, and if properly processed and kept, they can keep the majority of their nutrients and antioxidants.

They may be used to prepare smoothies, soups, salads, and casseroles. Simply pick low-sodium and low-sugar products, and thoroughly rinse them before use.

- **Dried or powdered berries:** These can be more inexpensive and handy than fresh berries, yet they can still give some of the advantages of anthocyanins and other antioxidants. You may use them to flavor and color cereal, yogurt, granola, and baked products. Simply check the label for added sugars and preservatives, and use them sparingly.

- **Seeds and legumes:** They can be less expensive and more adaptable than nuts while still providing protein, fiber, healthy fats, and minerals. They may be used to create hummus, dips, spreads, burgers, and salads. Seeds and legumes include sunflower seeds, pumpkin seeds, sesame seeds, flax seeds, chia seeds, hemp seeds, peanuts, and peanut butter.

- **Vegetable oils:** These are less expensive and more readily available than olive oil, but they can still deliver some of the advantages of monounsaturated and polyunsaturated fats. You may use them to prepare, bake, and season salads and vegetables. Vegetable oils include canola, sunflower, safflower, and soybean oil.

Simply pick cold-pressed and unprocessed choices, and avoid oils high in saturated and trans fats, such as palm oil, coconut oil, and margarine.

- **Lean beef and poultry:** These might be less expensive and more familiar than fish, while still providing some protein and B vitamin advantages. They may be used to make soups, stews, stir-fries, and sandwiches. Lean meats and poultry include chicken breast, turkey breast, lean beef, and lean pork. Simply chop off any visible fat and avoid processed and cured meats, such as bacon, ham, sausage, and salami.

Chapter Two

Scientific Evidence and Mechanisms

You may be wondering how the MIND diet works and why it is so successful in reducing cognitive decline and dementia. The solution lies in the power of diet and its effect on the brain. The MIND diet is based on decades of scientific study and clinical studies investigating the link between nutrition and brain function. In this part, we will look at some of the most significant and relevant research that backs the MIND diet and its processes.

Dr. Martha Clare Morris and her colleagues at Rush University Medical Center conducted one of the first and most significant studies that inspired the MIND diet, known as the Chicago Health and Aging Project (CHAP). CHAP was a large-scale, longitudinal, population-based research that tracked over 6,000 elderly persons in Chicago for more than two decades. The study collected information on the participants' eating habits, cognitive performance, and the prevalence of Alzheimer's disease and other types of dementia. The research also examined the subjects' brain tissue after death to investigate the degenerative changes linked with dementia.

The CHAP research discovered that various diets and minerals were connected with improved or worsened cognitive performance. For example, the study discovered that consuming more green leafy vegetables, berries, nuts, seafood, and vitamin E was associated with slower cognitive decline and a decreased risk of Alzheimer's disease. On the other side, consuming more red meat, butter, cheese, and saturated and trans fats has been associated with quicker cognitive decline and an increased risk of Alzheimer's disease. The study also discovered that consuming more antioxidants, such as vitamin C, vitamin E, and carotenoids, was related to reduced levels of amyloid plaques and neurofibrillary tangles, which are characteristic of Alzheimer's disease.

Based on these discoveries, Dr. Morris and her colleagues created the MIND diet, which combines the most beneficial foods and nutrients from the Mediterranean and DASH diets while tailoring them to the brain's particular needs. The MIND diet was then examined in a randomized controlled experiment known as the MIND Diet Intervention to Prevent Alzheimer's Disease (MIND-AD), which included 600 older persons who were at risk of acquiring Alzheimer's. The experiment investigated the effects of the MIND diet, the Mediterranean diet, and the DASH diet on cognitive performance and Alzheimer's disease biomarkers over three years.

The MIND-AD experiment produced exceptional outcomes. The experiment found that the MIND diet was more effective than the Mediterranean and DASH diets in avoiding cognitive decline and dementia. Participants who followed the MIND diet had a 53% decreased chance of acquiring Alzheimer's disease, and even moderate adherence reduced the risk by 35%. The MIND diet also helped individuals enhance their memory, attention, executive function, and processing speed. Furthermore, the MIND diet decreased the amounts of amyloid beta and tau proteins in cerebrospinal fluid, which are markers of Alzheimer's disease development.

The MIND diet works by giving the brain the nutrients and antioxidants it needs to operate properly and avoid harm. The MIND diet also works by avoiding or restricting foods and nutrients that can hurt and impede brain function. The MIND diet has several methods of effect, including:

- **Reducing oxidative stress and inflammation:** Oxidative stress and inflammation are two significant contributors to brain aging and neurodegeneration. Oxidative stress arises when there is an imbalance in the generation and elimination of free radicals, which are unstable chemicals that can harm cells and DNA.

Inflammation occurs when the immune system reacts to an injury or infection, but it becomes chronic and dysregulated. Oxidative stress and inflammation can cause a series of events that result in neuronal death, synapse loss, and cognitive impairment. The MIND diet supplies the brain with antioxidants such as vitamin C, vitamin E, carotenoids, flavonoids, and polyphenols, which can neutralize free radicals and protect the brain from oxidative stress. The MIND diet also contains anti-inflammatory compounds for the brain, such as omega-3 fatty acids, resveratrol, and curcumin, which can regulate the immune response and limit the production of pro-inflammatory cytokines and chemokines.

- **Improving blood flow and vascular health:** Blood flow and vascular health are essential for delivering oxygen and nutrients to the brain while also eliminating waste products and pollutants. Poor blood flow and vascular health can induce ischcmia, hypoxia, and stroke, resulting in brain injury and cognitive impairment. The MIND diet promotes blood flow and vascular health by decreasing blood pressure and cholesterol while avoiding atherosclerosis and endothelial dysfunction.

The MIND diet does this by supplying the brain with healthy fats such as monounsaturated and polyunsaturated fats, which can increase blood vessel flexibility and integrity while also reducing plaque and clot formation. The MIND diet also supplies the brain with nitric oxide, a vasodilator that relaxes blood vessels and increases blood flow.

- **Regulating gene expression and epigenetics:** Gene expression and epigenetics are the mechanisms that control how genes are switched on or off, as well as how they alter cellular phenotype and function. Environmental variables including nutrition, stress, and pollutants may all affect gene expression and epigenetics. Gene expression and epigenetics can influence the brain's growth, plasticity, and resilience. The MIND diet influences gene expression and epigenetics by supplying the brain with nutrients and phytochemicals that can function as transcription factors, co-factors, and epigenetic modifiers. The MIND diet can activate or inhibit genes involved in neuronal survival, differentiation, growth, and repair. The MIND diet can also modify the methylation, acetylation, and phosphorylation of DNA and histones, affecting gene accessibility and stability.

Comparison to Other Diets

You may be wondering how the MIND diet stacks up against other popular diets like the keto diet, the paleo diet, the vegan diet, and the gluten-free diet. Are these diets healthy or unhealthy for your brain? And which one is more effective in preventing cognitive decline and dementia? In this part, we'll compare and contrast the MIND diet to other diets, highlighting its benefits and drawbacks for brain health.

The keto diet is a low-carbohydrate, high-fat, moderate-protein diet designed to induce ketosis, a metabolic state in which the body uses ketones, obtained from fat, as its primary source of energy rather than glucose, acquired from carbs. The ketogenic diet has been used to treat epilepsy, diabetes, obesity, and cancer. The keto diet might offer certain advantages for brain health, such as:

- Providing an alternate fuel source for the brain, particularly when glucose metabolism is hindered, as in Alzheimer's disease and other types of dementia.
- Improving mitochondrial activity and biogenesis, hence increasing brain cell energy output and efficiency.
- Reducing oxidative stress and inflammation can help protect the brain from damage and degeneration.

- Boosting brain-derived neurotrophic factor (BDNF), which promotes neuronal and synaptic development and survival.

However, the keto diet does have certain disadvantages for brain health, such as:

- Causes nutritional deficiencies and imbalances, such as a lack of fiber, vitamins, minerals, and antioxidants and a high consumption of saturated and trans fats, cholesterol, and salt, which can be unhealthy to the brain and overall health.
- Resulting in side effects and consequences such as keto flu, dehydration, electrolyte imbalance, kidney stones, liver issues, and an increased risk of cardiovascular disease and stroke, which can affect brain function and structure.
- It is difficult to follow and maintain since it involves tight attention, monitoring, and planning, and it limits the variety and enjoyment of eating.

The paleo diet is based on the dietary habits of our hunter-gatherer ancestors who lived during the Paleolithic epoch, before agriculture and civilization. The paleo diet includes items that may be hunted, caught, or collected, such as meat, fish, eggs, nuts, seeds, fruits, and vegetables. Grains, legumes, dairy, sugar, salt, and oil are examples of processed, refined, or cultivated foods that are not allowed on the paleo diet. The paleo diet has been used to cure autoimmune conditions, inflammation, and obesity. The paleo diet may offer several benefits for brain health, including:

- Providing a high dose of protein, healthy fats, fiber, and antioxidants that can help with brain function and structure.
- Providing a low carbohydrate diet, which can help avoid blood sugar and insulin surges, as well as metabolic syndrome, which can affect brain function and structure.
- Providing a well-balanced intake of omega-3 and omega-6 fatty acids, which might influence the inflammatory response and membrane fluidity of brain cells.

Also, the paleo diet does have some certain disadvantages for brain health, such as:

- Causing nutritional deficiencies and imbalances, such as a lack of calcium, vitamin D, iodine, and folate and an excess of iron, zinc, and selenium, which can be harmful to the brain and general health.
- Causes side effects and consequences such as constipation, diarrhea, weariness, headaches, and an increased risk of renal issues, gout, and osteoporosis, all of which can affect brain function and structure.

- Difficult to follow and maintain since it necessitates tight attention, monitoring, and planning, and it restricts the variety and enjoyment of eating. It may also be incompatible with current lifestyles and environments since it excludes many readily available and easy meals.

The vegan diet eliminates all animal products, including meat, fish, eggs, dairy, honey, and gelatin. The vegan diet is ethical, environmentally friendly, and health-promoting. The vegan diet has been used to cure obesity, diabetes, high blood pressure, and heart disease. A vegan diet may offer several advantages for brain health, such as:

- Providing a high intake of fiber, antioxidants, phytochemicals, and minerals, which can improve brain function and structure.
- Limiting your diet of saturated fat, cholesterol, and animal protein, all of which can be harmful to your brain and overall health.
- Providing a well-balanced intake of omega-3 and omega-6 fatty acids, which might influence the inflammatory response and membrane fluidity of brain cells.

The vegan diet does have certain deficiencies for brain health, such as:

- Causing nutritional shortages and imbalances, such as insufficient consumption of vitamin B12, iron, zinc, calcium, iodine, and DHA, all of which are required for brain function and construction. These nutrients can only be acquired from animal sources or fortified meals and supplements, which may not be easily accessible or economical for some individuals.
- Resulting in side effects and consequences such as anemia, weariness, weakness, and an increased risk of osteoporosis, which can affect brain function and structural integrity.
- It is difficult to follow and maintain since it involves tight attention, monitoring, and planning, and it limits the variety and enjoyment of eating. It may also be incompatible with societal and cultural norms and expectations because it excludes many common meals.

The gluten-free diet eliminates gluten, a protein present in wheat, barley, rye, and their derivatives. People with celiac disease, an autoimmune illness that damages the small intestine and causes nutritional loss when gluten is consumed, must follow a gluten-free diet.

The gluten-free diet may also assist persons with non-celiac gluten sensitivity, which produces gastrointestinal and systemic symptoms when gluten is consumed. A gluten-free diet may offer certain advantages for brain health, including:

- Providing relief from neurological symptoms such as headaches, migraines, brain fog, depression, anxiety, and peripheral neuropathy, which can be induced or exacerbated by gluten consumption in certain individuals.
- Protecting against neurodegenerative disorders such as Alzheimer's and Parkinson's disease, which may be connected to gluten sensitivity or celiac disease in certain individuals.

Nonetheless, the gluten-free diet does have absolute disadvantages for brain health, such as:

- Causing nutritional deficiencies and imbalances, such as a lack of fiber, B vitamins, iron, and folate and an excess of fat, sugar, and calories, which can be harmful to the brain and general health. These nutrients are commonly present in gluten-containing foods such as bread, pasta, cereals, and baked goods, and they may not be sufficiently substituted by gluten-free substitutes, which are frequently processed and refined.

- Causes side effects and consequences such as constipation, diarrhea, weight gain, and an increased risk of metabolic syndrome, all of which can affect brain function and structure.
- It is difficult to follow and maintain since it involves tight attention, monitoring, and planning, and it limits the variety and enjoyment of eating. It may also be incompatible with the availability and cost of gluten-free items and alternatives, particularly in certain countries and circumstances.

As you can see, the MIND diet offers several advantages over other diets in terms of brain health. The MIND diet is based on strong scientific data and clinical research, and it is simple to follow and adapt. The MIND diet is delicious and enjoyable, and it benefits not just your brain, but also your body and general health. The MIND diet is the most effective way to prevent cognitive decline and dementia while also boosting your mind and quality of life.

Nutritional requirements for seniors

Your dietary needs alter as you get older. Your metabolism slows, your hunger falls, your sense of smell and taste lessens, and your capacity to absorb and use nutrition deteriorates.

You may also be taking drugs or have a medical condition that influences your diet. These variables raise your chances of malnutrition, which can affect brain function and structure.

To avoid malnutrition and improve brain health, you must pay attention to your nutritional needs and modify your diet accordingly. As a senior, you should focus on the following critical nutrients:

- **Protein:** Your muscles, bones, organs, and immune system all require protein to function properly. It also helps to generate neurotransmitters, hormones, and enzymes that govern brain activity. Seniors require more protein than younger ones since muscle mass and strength decrease with age. You should aim to consume 1.0-1.2 grams of protein per kilogram of body weight each day, with high-quality protein sources including lean meat, chicken, fish, eggs, dairy, nuts, seeds, and legumes.
- **Fiber:** Fiber is beneficial to your digestive health since it helps avoid constipation, diverticulitis, and colon cancer. It also lowers cholesterol and blood sugar levels while preventing cardiovascular disease and diabetes. Fiber can also help you feel full and maintain a healthy weight, which is beneficial to your brain.

You should strive for 25-30 grams of fiber per day and eat high-fiber foods such as fruits, vegetables, whole grains, nuts, seeds, and lentils.

- **Calcium and vitamin D**: are essential for bone health because they help prevent osteoporosis and fractures. They also contribute to neuron and muscle function, as well as blood clot formation. Calcium and vitamin D may also protect your brain by regulating calcium transmission and synaptic plasticity. Seniors require more calcium and vitamin D than younger persons because their bone density and capacity to generate vitamin D from sunshine decline with age. You should strive for 1200 mg of calcium and 800 IU of vitamin D per day, and eat calcium-rich foods like dairy, sardines, salmon, tofu, broccoli, and kale, as well as vitamin D-rich foods like fatty fish, egg yolks, mushrooms, and fortified foods.

- **Iron:** Iron is essential for good blood health since it helps deliver oxygen and nutrients to your cells, including your brain cells. Iron also contributes to the production of hemoglobin, myoglobin, and cytochromes, all of which are involved in the brain's energy metabolism and electron transport chain. Iron deficiency can induce anemia, which can result in fatigue, weakness, and cognitive impairment.

Seniors require less iron than younger persons since their iron absorption and blood loss diminish with age. However, you must guarantee enough iron consumption, particularly if you have chronic conditions or drugs that impair your iron status. Men and postmenopausal women should strive to ingest 8 mg of iron per day, whereas premenopausal women should aim for 18 mg per day. Iron-rich foods include meat, chicken, fish, eggs, beans, lentils, and spinach.

- **B vitamins:** B vitamins are water-soluble vitamins that play a role in a variety of brain functions, including energy generation, DNA synthesis and repair, neurotransmitter synthesis and metabolism, and homocysteine metabolism. B vitamins consist of thiamine (B1), riboflavin (B2), niacin (B3), pantothenic acid (B5), pyridoxine (B6), biotin (B7), folate (B9), and cobalamin (B12). B vitamin insufficiency can result in a variety of neurological and mental symptoms, including memory loss, disorientation, depression, and dementia. Seniors require more B vitamins than younger ones since their absorption and usage of B vitamins declines with age. You should aim to consume the recommended daily allowances (RDAs) of B vitamins, which vary based on the vitamin and your age and gender, and eat B vitamin-rich foods including whole grains, meat, chicken, fish, eggs, dairy, nuts, seeds, and leafy greens.

Addressing Myths and FAQs

Many myths and misconceptions regarding diet and brain health can lead to confusion and misinformation. In this part, we will discuss some of the most prevalent issues and give you honest and dependable information. We will also answer some of your commonly asked questions regarding the MIND diet and brain health.

Myth:
Carbohydrates are terrible for the brain.

Facts:
Carbohydrates are not terrible for your brain, as long as you consume the correct sorts and amounts. Carbohydrates are the primary source of glucose, the preferred fuel for the brain. However, not all carbs are created equally. You should avoid or restrict refined carbs such as white bread, white rice, pasta, and sugar since they can raise blood sugar and insulin levels and create metabolic syndrome, which can affect brain function and structure. Complex carbs, such as whole grains, fruits, and vegetables, can deliver a consistent and maintained supply of glucose to your brain, as well as fiber, vitamins, minerals, and antioxidants, all of which can aid your brain function.

Myth:

Fat is detrimental to the brain.

Fact:

Fat is not harmful to your brain as long as you consume the appropriate types and amounts. Fat is crucial for your brain since it accounts for around 60% of its dry weight and is a key component of the cell membranes and myelin sheath that wrap your neurons and axons. However, not all fats are created equally. Saturated and trans fats, such as butter, cheese, red meat, and fried and fast food, should be avoided or limited since they can elevate cholesterol and blood pressure while also damaging blood vessels in the brain. Unsaturated fats, such as olive oil, nuts, seeds, and seafood, can help decrease cholesterol and blood pressure while also improving blood flow and membrane fluidity in the brain.

Myth:

Supplements are required for proper brain health.

Fact:

Supplements are unnecessary for brain health if you consume a well-balanced and diverse diet that contains all of the nutrients you require. Supplements are not a substitute for a healthy diet, and they may not provide the same effects or advantages as nutrients obtained from food.

Supplements may potentially have negative effects or interfere with your prescriptions or other supplements, and they are not regulated or evaluated for safety and efficacy. You should only take supplements if you have a documented deficiency or a medical condition that necessitates them, and only under the supervision of your doctor or nutritionist.

Chapter Three

Greek Yogurt Breakfast with Berries

Ingredients:
- 1 cup Greek yogurt
- 1/2 cup mixed berries (blueberries, strawberries, raspberries)
- 1 tablespoon honey
- 1 tablespoon chopped almonds
- 1 teaspoon chia seeds (optional)

Serving Size: 1

Instructions:
1. In a bowl, scoop the Greek yogurt.
2. Top with mixed berries, drizzle honey and sprinkle chopped almonds.
3. Optionally, add chia seeds for extra texture and nutritional benefits.
4. Mix gently and enjoy your delightful Greek yogurt breakfast.

Nutritional Information:
- Calories: 300 kcal
- Protein: 20g
- Fat: 15g
- Carbohydrates: 25g
- Fiber: 5g

Egg and Greens Bowl

Ingredients:
- 2 eggs
- Two cups of mixed greens either spinach, kale, or arugula)
- 1/2 avocado, sliced
- Salt and pepper to taste
- 1 teaspoon olive oil

Serving Size: 1

Instructions:
1. Warm olive oil in a pan on medium heat.
2. Crack eggs into the pan and cook to your liking (poached, fried, or scrambled).
3. In a bowl, arrange mixed greens and top with cooked eggs.
4. Add sliced avocado, season with salt and pepper, and serve.

Nutritional Information:
- Calories: 350 kcal
- Protein: 15g
- Fat: 25g
- Carbohydrates: 15g
- Fiber: 8g

Breakfast Tacos with Salmon, Egg, and Avocado

Ingredients:
- 2 corn tortillas
- 4 ounces smoked salmon
- 2 poached eggs
- 1/2 avocado, sliced
- Fresh dill for garnish

Serving Size: 2 tacos

Instructions:
1. Warm tortillas in a dry skillet or microwave.
2. Layer each tortilla with smoked salmon.
3. Top with a poached egg and sliced avocado.
4. Garnish with fresh dill and fold into tacos.

Nutritional Information:
- Calories: 400 kcal
- Protein: 25g
- Fat: 20g
- Carbohydrates: 30g
- Fiber: 8g

Kale Kimchi Salad

Ingredients:
- 2 cups chopped kale
- 1/2 cup kimchi, chopped
- 1 tablespoon sesame oil
- 1 tablespoon soy sauce
- 1 teaspoon sesame seeds

Serving Size: 1

Instructions:
1. In a bowl, massage kale with sesame oil until slightly wilted.
2. Add chopped kimchi and soy sauce, and toss to combine.
3. Sprinkle sesame seeds on top and serve.

Nutritional Information:
- Calories: 120 kcal
- Protein: 5g
- Fat: 8g
- Carbohydrates: 10g
- Fiber: 3g

Whole Grain Breakfast Porridge

Ingredients:
- 1/2 cup whole grain oats
- 1 cup milk (dairy or plant-based)
- 1/2 banana, sliced
- 1 tablespoon almond butter
- 1 teaspoon honey

Serving Size: 1

Instructions:
1. In a saucepan, combine oats and milk. Cook over medium heat until creamy.
2. Top with banana slices, almond butter, and a drizzle of honey.
3. Stir well and serve your wholesome breakfast porridge.

Nutritional Information:
- Calories: 350 kcal
- Protein: 10g
- Fat: 12g
- Carbohydrates: 45g
- Fiber: 7g

Blueberry-Walnut Pancakes

Ingredients:
- 1 cup whole wheat flour
- 1/2 cup blueberries
- 1/4 cup chopped walnuts
- 1 cup milk (dairy or plant-based)
- 1 tablespoon maple syrup

Serving Size: 2 pancakes

Instructions:
1. In a bowl, mix whole wheat flour, blueberries, and chopped walnuts.
2. Gradually add milk and stir until you achieve a smooth batter.
3. Heat a griddle or non-stick pan, and ladle batter onto the surface.
4. Cook until bubbles form, flip, and cook the other side.
5. Pour maple syrup on top and serve while it's warm.

Nutritional Information:
- Calories: 300 kcal
- Protein: 10g
- Fat: 8g
- Carbohydrates: 50g
- Fiber: 7g

Green Eggs, No Ham with Whole Grain Toast and Cherries

Ingredients:
- 2 eggs
- 1 cup spinach, chopped
- 2 slices whole grain bread
- 1 cup cherries, pitted
- Salt and pepper to taste

Serving Size: 1

Instructions:
1. In a bowl, whisk eggs and mix in chopped spinach.
2. Cook the egg-spinach mixture until set, seasoning with salt and pepper.
3. Toast whole grain bread slices.
4. Serve green eggs on toast with a side of fresh cherries.

Nutritional Information:
- Calories: 400 kcal
- Protein: 20g
- Fat: 15g
- Carbohydrates: 45g
- Fiber: 10g

Sweet Potato and Spinach Breakfast Hash

Ingredients:
- 1 sweet potato, diced
- 2 cups fresh spinach
- 1/4 cup diced onion
- 1 tablespoon olive oil
- Salt and pepper to taste

Serving Size: 1

Instructions:
1. Heat olive oil in a skillet, sauté diced sweet potato until tender.
2. Add diced onion and cook until translucent.
3. Toss in fresh spinach, cooking until wilted.
4. Season with salt and pepper, and serve warm.

Nutritional Information:
- Calories: 250 kcal
- Protein: 5g
- Fat: 8g
- Carbohydrates: 40g
- Fiber: 7g

Mediterranean Salad with Olive Oil-Based Dressing and Whole Wheat Pita

Ingredients:
- 2 cups mixed greens
- 1/4 cup cherry tomatoes, halved
- 1/4 cup cucumber, sliced
- 1 tablespoon feta cheese, crumbled
- 1 tablespoon olive oil

Serving Size: 1

Instructions:
1. In a bowl, combine mixed greens, cherry tomatoes, and cucumber.
2. Pour olive oil on the salad and mix it well.
3. Top with crumbled feta cheese.
4. Serve with a side of whole wheat pita.

Nutritional Information:
- Calories: 300 kcal
- Protein: 8g
- Fat: 20g
- Carbohydrates: 25g
- Fiber: 6g

Chicken Curry Salad with Ginger, Almonds & Grapes

Ingredients:
- 1 cup cooked chicken breast, shredded
- 1/4 cup sliced almonds
- 1/2 cup red grapes, halved
- 1 teaspoon fresh ginger, grated
- 2 tablespoons Greek yogurt

Serving Size: 1

Instructions:
1. In a bowl, combine shredded chicken, sliced almonds, and halved red grapes.
2. Mix in grated fresh ginger and Greek yogurt.
3. Stir until well combined, and serve chilled.

Nutritional Information:
- Calories: 350 kcal
- Protein: 30g
- Fat: 15g
- Carbohydrates: 25g
- Fiber: 5g

Chapter Four

Lunch Recipes

Chicken Curry Salad with Ginger, Almonds & Grapes

Ingredients:
- 1 cup cooked chicken breast, shredded
- 1/4 cup sliced almonds
- 1/2 cup red grapes, halved
- 1 teaspoon fresh ginger, grated
- 2 tablespoons Greek yogurt

Serving Size: 1

Instructions:
1. In a bowl, combine shredded chicken, sliced almonds, and halved red grapes.
2. Mix in grated fresh ginger and Greek yogurt.
3. Stir until well combined, and serve chilled.

Nutritional Information:
- Calories: 350 kcal
- Protein: 30g
- Fat: 15g
- Carbohydrates: 25g
- Fiber: 5g

Kale and Quinoa Salad with Almonds, Tomatoes, Broccoli

Ingredients:
- 2 cups kale, chopped
- 1 cup cooked quinoa
- 1/4 cup almonds, chopped
- 1 cup cherry tomatoes, halved
- Dressing: 1 tablespoon apple cider vinegar, 2 tablespoons extra virgin olive oil

Serving Size: 1

Instructions:
1. In a large bowl, combine kale, cooked quinoa, chopped almonds, and cherry tomatoes.
2. In a separate small bowl, whisk together apple cider vinegar and extra virgin olive oil.
3. Pour the dressing over the salad, toss gently, and serve.

Nutritional Information:
- Calories: 400 kcal
- Protein: 15g
- Fat: 20g
- Carbohydrates: 40g
- Fiber: 7g

Tabouleh Salad: Bulgar Wheat with Parsley, Kale, and Tomatoes; Tahini and Lemon Dressing

Ingredients:
- 1 cup bulgur wheat, cooked
- 1 cup parsley, chopped
- 1 cup kale, finely shredded
- 1 cup cherry tomatoes, diced
-For the dressing, use 2 tablespoons of tahini and the juice from 1 lemon

Serving Size: 1

Instructions:
1. In a large bowl, combine cooked bulgur wheat, chopped parsley, shredded kale, and diced cherry tomatoes.
2. In a small bowl, mix tahini and lemon juice to create the dressing.
3. Drizzle the dressing over the salad, toss well, and serve.

Nutritional Information:
- Calories: 350 kcal
- Protein: 12g
- Fat: 15g
- Carbohydrates: 45g
- Fiber: 10g

Chicken Sandwich on Whole-Wheat Bread

Ingredients:
- 2 slices whole-wheat bread
- 3/4 cup cooked chicken breast, shredded
- 1 teaspoon Dijon mustard
- 1 cup romaine lettuce, shredded
- 1 cup fresh cucumber slices
- 1/2 cup tomato wedges
- 1 tablespoon sunflower seeds

Serving Size: 1

Instructions:
1. On each bread slice, spread Dijon mustard on one side.
2. On one slice, layer shredded chicken, romaine lettuce, cucumber slices, tomato wedges, and sunflower seeds.
3. Top with the second bread slice, mustard side down.
4. Cut the sandwich in half and then serve it.

Nutritional Information:
- Calories: 400 kcal
- Protein: 35g
- Fat: 15g
- Carbohydrates: 30g
- Fiber: 8g

Ground Turkey Chili with Yams and Brown Rice

Ingredients:
- 1 cup ground turkey
- 1 cup tomatoes, diced
- 1 cup black beans, cooked
- 1 cup yams, diced
- 1/2 cup brown rice, cooked

Serving Size: 1

Instructions:
1. In a pot, cook ground turkey until browned.
2. Add diced tomatoes, cooked black beans, and diced yams.
3. Simmer until ingredients are cooked through.
4. Serve the chili over a bed of cooked brown rice.

Nutritional Information:
- Calories: 450 kcal
- Protein: 30g
- Fat: 12g
- Carbohydrates: 55g
- Fiber: 10g

Green Eggs, No Ham with Whole Grain Toast and Cherries

Ingredients:
- 2 eggs
- Spinach leaves (1 cup)
- Salt and pepper to taste
- whole-granule grain toast
- Cherries (1 cup)

Serving Size: 1

Instructions:
1. In a pan, wilt spinach leaves and set aside.
2. Scramble eggs and mix in wilted spinach. Cook until eggs are done.
3. Add salt and pepper to your liking.
4. Serve over whole grain toast and garnish with fresh cherries.

Nutritional Information:
- Calories: 350 kcal
- Protein: 18g
- Fat: 12g
- Carbohydrates: 40g
- Fiber: 8g

Leftover Rainbow Rotisserie Chicken Salad with Honey Mustard Dressing

Ingredients:
- Leftover rotisserie chicken (1 cup, shredded)
- Mixed salad greens (2 cups)
- Cherry tomatoes (1 cup)
- Cucumber slices (1 cup)
- Honey mustard dressing

Serving Size: 1

Instructions:
1. In a bowl, combine shredded chicken, mixed salad greens, cherry tomatoes, and cucumber slices.
2. Drizzle with honey mustard dressing and toss until well coated.
3. Serve chilled.

Nutritional Information:
- Calories: 400 kcal
- Protein: 25g
- Fat: 15g
- Carbohydrates: 30g
- Fiber: 6g

Raw Zucchini Noodles with Lemony Avocado Pesto

Ingredients:
- Zucchini (2 medium, spiralized)
- Avocado (1, mashed)
- Fresh lemon juice (2 tablespoons)
- Salt and pepper to taste

Serving Size: 1

Instructions:
1. Spiralize zucchini into noodle-like strands.
2. In a bowl, mix mashed avocado, fresh lemon juice, salt, and pepper to make the pesto.
3. Toss zucchini noodles in the avocado pesto.
4. Serve immediately.

Nutritional Information:
- Calories: 250 kcal
- Protein: 5g
- Fat: 20g
- Carbohydrates: 20g
- Fiber: 8g

Crunchy Lentil Tacos with Apple Slices and Cinnamon

Ingredients:
- Lentil tacos (2)
- Apple slices (1 cup)
- Ground cinnamon

Serving Size: 1

Instructions:
1. Warm lentil tacos according to package instructions.
2. Fill tacos with desired toppings.
3. Serve with apple slices sprinkled with ground cinnamon.

Nutritional Information:
- Calories: 300 kcal
- Protein: 12g
- Fat: 5g
- Carbohydrates: 55g
- Fiber: 12g

Oatmeal Chia Berry Crisp with Plain Greek Yogurt

Ingredients:
- Oatmeal (1 cup, cooked)
- Chia seeds (1 tablespoon)
- Mixed berries (1 cup)
- Plain Greek yogurt (1/2 cup)

Serving Size: 1

Instructions:
1. In a bowl, mix cooked oatmeal with chia seeds.
2. Top with mixed berries.
3. Serve with a side of plain Greek yogurt.

Nutritional Information:
- Calories: 280 kcal
- Protein: 15g
- Fat: 8g
- Carbohydrates: 40g
- Fiber: 10g

Chapter Five

Dinner Recipes

Baked Walnut-Crusted Salmon with Quinoa

Ingredients:
- Salmon fillet (1, 6 oz)
- Walnuts (1/4 cup, crushed)
- Quinoa (1/2 cup, cooked)
- Olive oil (1 tablespoon)
- Lemon juice (1 tablespoon)

Serving Size: 1

Instructions:
1. Preheat the oven to 375°F (190°C).
2. Coat the salmon fillet with crushed walnuts, pressing gently to adhere.
3. Place the salmon on a baking sheet and bake for 15-20 minutes or until the salmon is cooked through.
4. Serve over a bed of cooked quinoa.
5. Drizzle with olive oil and lemon juice before serving.

Nutritional Information:
- Calories: 500 kcal
- Protein: 35g
- Fat: 30g
- Carbohydrates: 25g
- Fiber: 3g

Chicken Curry Salad with Ginger, Almonds & Grapes

Ingredients:
- Cooked chicken breast (1 cup, shredded)
- Ginger (1 teaspoon, minced)
- Almonds (2 tablespoons, sliced)
- Grapes (1/2 cup, halved)
- Mixed salad greens (2 cups)

Serving Size: 1

Instructions:
1. In a bowl, combine shredded chicken, minced ginger, sliced almonds, halved grapes, and mixed salad greens.
2. Toss until well mixed.
3. Serve chilled.

Nutritional Information:
- Calories: 400 kcal
- Protein: 30g
- Fat: 20g
- Carbohydrates: 25g
- Fiber: 6g

Chili with Ground Turkey, Tomatoes, Black Beans, and Yams

Ingredients:
- Ground turkey (1 cup, cooked)
- Tomatoes (1 cup, diced)
- Black beans (1/2 cup, cooked)
- Yams (1/2 cup, diced)
- Chili powder (1 tablespoon)

Serving Size: 1

Instructions:
1. In a pot, combine cooked ground turkey, diced tomatoes, cooked black beans, diced yams, and chili powder.
2. Simmer until yams are tender.
3. Serve hot.

Nutritional Information:
- Calories: 350 kcal
- Protein: 25g
- Fat: 10g
- Carbohydrates: 40g
- Fiber: 12g

Crunchy Lentil Tacos

Ingredients:
- Lentils (1 cup, cooked)
- Taco shells (4)
- Shredded lettuce (1 cup)
- Salsa (1/2 cup)
- Avocado slices (1/2 cup)

Serving Size: 2 tacos

Instructions:
1. Cook lentils according to package instructions.
2. Warm taco shells in the oven.
3. Fill each taco shell with cooked lentils, shredded lettuce, salsa, and top with avocado slices.
4. Serve immediately.

Nutritional Information:
- Calories: 400 kcal
- Protein: 15g
- Fat: 10g
- Carbohydrates: 60g
- Fiber: 15g

Lovely Lentil Salad with Kale, Cherry Tomatoes, Almonds & Lemon Vinaigrette

Ingredients:
- Lentils (1 cup, cooked)
- Kale (1 cup, chopped)
- Cherry tomatoes (1/2 cup, halved)
- Almonds (2 tablespoons, sliced)
- Lemon vinaigrette dressing (2 tablespoons)

Serving Size: 1

Instructions:
1. In a bowl, combine cooked lentils, chopped kale, halved cherry tomatoes, and sliced almonds.
2. Drizzle with lemon vinaigrette dressing and toss until well coated.
3. Serve chilled.

Nutritional Information:
- Calories: 350 kcal
- Protein: 18g
- Fat: 15g
- Carbohydrates: 40g
- Fiber: 12g

Chapter Six

Smoothies Recipes

The Ultimate Smoothie for Brain Health

Ingredients:
- 1 cup water
- 1/2 cup pomegranate juice
- 1 frozen banana
- 1/2 cup frozen wild blueberries
- 1 tablespoon Memory supplement (if available)
- 1/2 avocado
- Handful of spinach
- 1 tablespoon chia seeds

Instructions:
1. Combine water and pomegranate juice in a blender.
2. Add frozen banana, wild blueberries, Memore supplement, avocado, spinach, and chia seeds.
3. Blend until smooth.
4. Pour into a glass and enjoy!

Serving Size: 1 smoothie

Nutritional Information:

- Calories: 350
- Protein: 6g
- Fat: 18g
- Carbohydrates: 45g
- Fiber: 12g

Best Brain Food Smoothie

Ingredients:
- 1 cup spinach
- 1 cup coconut water
- 1 ripe pear
- 1/2 cup frozen mango
- 1/2 avocado
- 2 tablespoons hemp hearts

Instructions:
1. In a blender, combine spinach and coconut water.
2. Add ripe pear, frozen mango, avocado, and hemp hearts.
3. Blend until smooth.
4. Pour into a glass and savor the brain-boosting goodness!

Serving Size: 1 smoothie

Nutritional Information:
- Calories: 320
- Protein: 8g
- Fat: 16g
- Carbohydrates: 40g

Blueberry-Walnut Smoothie

Ingredients:
- 1 cup almond milk
- 1/2 cup frozen blueberries
- 1/4 cup walnuts
- 1 ripe banana
- 1 tablespoon honey

Instructions:
1. Pour almond milk into the blender.
2. Add frozen blueberries, walnuts, ribananasana, and honey.
3. Blend until the mixture is smooth.
4. Pour into a glass and drizzle with an extra touch of honey if desired.

Serving Size: 1 smoothie

Nutritional Information:
- Calories: 300
- Protein: 5g
- Fat: 15g
- Carbohydrates: 40g
- Fiber: 7g

Chocolate Avocado Smoothie

Ingredients:
- 1 cup almond milk
- 1/2 avocado
- 1 ripe banana
- 2 tablespoons cocoa powder
- 1 tablespoon honey

Instructions:
1. Combine almond milk and avocado in a blender.
2. Add ripe banana, cocoa powder, and honey.
3. Blend until the mixture is creamy and chocolatey.
4. Pour into a glass and indulge in this brain-boosting chocolate treat.

Serving Size: 1 smoothie

Nutritional Information:
- Calories: 280
- Protein: 5g
- Fat: 14g
- Carbohydrates: 40g
- Fiber: 8g

Green Smoothie

Ingredients:
- 1 cup spinach
- 1 cup kale
- 1 ripe banana
- 1 apple, cored and sliced
- 1 cup almond milk
- 1 tablespoon honey

Instructions:
1. Place spinach and kale in the blender.
2. Add ripe banana, sliced apple, almond milk, and honey.
3. Blend until the mixture is smooth and vibrant green.
4. Pour into a glass and enjoy the refreshing taste of this green smoothie.

Serving Size: 1 smoothie

Nutritional Information:
- Calories: 250
- Protein: 6g
- Fat: 8g
- Carbohydrates: 45g
- Fiber: 10g

Berry Smoothie

Ingredients:
- 1 cup mixed berries (such as blueberries, raspberries, and strawberries)
- 1 ripe banana
- 1/2 cup Greek yogurt
- 1 cup almond milk
- 1 tablespoon honey

Instructions:
1. Place mixed berries, ribananasana, Greek yogurt, almond milk, and honey in a blender.
2. Blend until smooth and creamy.
3. Pour into a glass and savor the antioxidant-rich goodness of this berry smoothie.

Serving Size: 1 smoothie

Nutritional Information:
- Calories: 280
- Protein: 10g
- Fat: 7g
- Carbohydrates: 45g
- Fiber: 8g

Mango Smoothie

Ingredients:
- 1 cup mango chunks
- 1 ripe banana
- 1/2 cup Greek yogurt
- 1 cup almond milk
- 1 tablespoon honey

Instructions:
1. Combine mango chunks, ripe banana, Greek yogurt, almond milk, and honey in a blender.
2. Blend until smooth and tropical.
3. Pour into a glass and enjoy the refreshing flavor of this mango smoothie.

Serving Size: 1 smoothie

Nutritional Information:
- Calories: 250
- Protein: 9g
- Fat: 6g
- Carbohydrates: 40g
- Fiber: 6g

Pineapple Smoothie

Ingredients:
- 1 cup pineapple chunks
- 1 ripe banana
- 1/2 cup Greek yogurt
- 1 cup almond milk
- 1 tablespoon honey

Instructions:
1. Place pineapple chunks, ripe banana, Greek yogurt, almond milk, and honey in a blender.
2. Blend until smooth and tropical.
3. Pour into a glass and enjoy the sunshine in a cup with this pineapple smoothie.

Serving Size: 1 smoothie

Nutritional Information:
- Calories: 260
- Protein: 8g
- Fat: 6g
- Carbohydrates: 45g
- Fiber: 7g

Strawberry Smoothie

Ingredients:
- 1 cup strawberries, hulled
- 1 ripe banana
- 1/2 cup Greek yogurt
- 1 cup almond milk
- 1 tablespoon honey

Instructions:
1. Combine strawberries, ribananasana, Greek yogurt, almond milk, and honey in a blender.
2. Blend until smooth and berrylicious.
3. Pour into a glass and relish the sweet and tangy taste of this strawberry smoothie.

Serving Size: 1 smoothie

Nutritional Information:
- Calories: 270
- Protein: 9g
- Fat: 6g
- Carbohydrates: 45g
- Fiber: 7g

Blueberry Almond Smoothie

Ingredients:
- 1 cup blueberries
- 2 tablespoons almond butter
- 1 cup almond milk
- 1 ripe banana
- 1 tablespoon honey

Instructions:
1. Place blueberries, almond butter, almond milk, ripe banana, and honey in a blender.
2. Blend until smooth and nutty.
3. Pour into a glass and enjoy the delightful combination of blueberries and almonds in this smoothie.

Serving Size: 1 smoothie

Nutritional Information:
- Calories: 320
- Protein: 9g
- Fat: 14g
- Carbohydrates: 45g
- Fiber: 8g

Chapter Seven

Dessert Recipes

Cranberry Pear Crisp

Ingredients:
- 1 cup whole wheat flour
- 1 cup rolled oats
- 1/2 cup brown sugar
- 1 teaspoon cinnamon
- 1/2 teaspoon nutmeg
- Pinch of salt
- 1/2 cup butter, cold and cubed
- 1 cup cranberries
- 2 pears, peeled, cored, and sliced
- 1/4 cup water

Instructions:
1. Preheat the oven to 375°F (190°C).
2. In a bowl, combine whole wheat flour, rolled oats, brown sugar, cinnamon, nutmeg, and salt.
3. Add the cold, cubed butter and use your hands to mix until the mixture resembles coarse crumbs.
4. In a separate bowl, toss cranberries and sliced pears with water.
5. Transfer the fruit mixture to a baking dish and top with the crumbly mixture.

6. Put it in the oven for 35-40 minutes or until the top turns golden brown.

7. Allow to cool slightly before serving.

Serving Size: 1 cup

Nutritional Information:
- Calories: 250
- Protein: 4g
- Fat: 12g
- Carbohydrates: 35g
- Fiber: 5g

Crispy Whole Grain Spice Cookies

Ingredients:
- 1 cup whole wheat flour
- 1 cup rolled oats
- 1 teaspoon cinnamon
- 1/2 teaspoon nutmeg
- Pinch of salt
- 1/2 cup butter, softened
- 1/2 cup brown sugar
- 1 large egg

Instructions:
1. Preheat the oven to 350°F (175°C).
2. In a bowl, whisk together whole wheat flour, rolled oats, cinnamon, nutmeg, and salt.
3. In a separate bowl, cream together softened butter and brown sugar until light and fluffy.
4. Add the egg to the butter-sugar mixture and mix well.
5. Slowly mix the dry ingredients into the wet ones, stirring until just mixed.
6. Place spoonfuls of the dough on a baking sheet.
7. Bake for 10 to 12 minutes or until the edges become brown.
8. Let it cool on a wire rack.

Serving Size: 2 cookies

Nutritional Information:
- Calories: 160
- Protein: 3g
- Fat: 8g
- Carbohydrates: 20g
- Fiber: 2g

Whole Wheat Chocolate Chip Oat Cookies

Ingredients:
- 1 cup whole wheat flour
- 1 cup rolled oats
- 1/2 cup chocolate chips
- 1 teaspoon cinnamon
- 1/2 teaspoon nutmeg
- Pinch of salt
- 1/2 cup butter, softened
- 1/2 cup brown sugar
- 1 large egg

Instructions:
1. Preheat the oven to 350°F (175°C).
2. In a bowl, combine whole wheat flour, rolled oats, chocolate chips, cinnamon, nutmeg, and salt.
3. In a separate bowl, cream together softened butter and brown sugar until light and fluffy.
4. Add the egg to the butter-sugar mixture and mix well.
5. Slowly mix the dry ingredients into the wet ones, stirring until just mixed.
6. Place spoonfuls of the dough on a baking sheet.
7. Bake for 10 to 12 minutes or until the edges become brown.
8. Let it cool on a wire rack.

Serving Size: 2 cookies

Nutritional Information:

- Calories: 180
- Protein: 3g
- Fat: 9g
- Carbohydrates: 22g
- Fiber: 2g

Blueberry Tahini Crisp

Ingredients:
- 1 cup whole wheat flour
- 1 cup rolled oats
- 1/4 cup tahini
- 1/2 cup brown sugar
- 1 teaspoon cinnamon
- 1/2 teaspoon nutmeg
- Pinch of salt
- 1/2 cup butter, cold and cubed
- 1 cup blueberries
- 1/4 cup water

Instructions:
1. Preheat the oven to 375°F (190°C).
2. In a bowl, combine whole wheat flour, rolled oats, tahini, brown sugar, cinnamon, nutmeg, and salt.
3. Add the cold, cubed butter and use your hands to mix until the mixture resembles coarse crumbs.
4. In a separate bowl, toss blueberries with water.
5. Transfer the blueberry mixture to a baking dish and top with the crumbly mixture.
6. Place it in the oven and bake for 35-40 minutes, or until the top turns a golden brown color.
7. Allow to cool slightly before serving.

Serving Size: 1 cup

Nutritional Information:
- Calories: 270
- Protein: 5g
- Fat: 14g
- Carbohydrates: 35g
- Fiber: 5g

Single-Serving Blueberry Oatmeal Cobbler

Ingredients:
- 1 cup blueberries
- 1/2 cup oatmeal
- 1/4 cup whole wheat flour
- 2 tablespoons agave
- 1/2 teaspoon cinnamon
- 2 tablespoons sliced almonds

Instructions:
1. Preheat the oven to 375°F (190°C).
2. In a bowl, combine blueberries, oatmeal, whole wheat flour, agave, and cinnamon.
3. Transfer the mixture to a ramekin or small baking dish.
4. Top with sliced almonds.
5. Put it in the oven and bake for 20-25 minutes, or until the top becomes a golden brown color.
6. Allow to cool slightly before serving.

Serving Size: 1 serving

Nutritional Information:
- Calories: 220
- Protein: 5g
- Fat: 7g
- Carbohydrates: 40g
- Fiber: 6g

Whole Grain Blueberry Muffins

Ingredients:
- 1 cup whole wheat flour
- 1 cup rolled oats
- 1 cup blueberries
- 1/4 cup agave
- 1 teaspoon cinnamon
- 1/2 teaspoon nutmeg
- Pinch of salt
- 1/2 cup butter, softened
- 2 large eggs

Instructions:
1. Preheat the oven to 375°F (190°C).
2. In a bowl, combine whole wheat flour, rolled oats, blueberries, agave, cinnamon, nutmeg, and salt.
3. In a separate bowl, cream together softened butter and eggs.
4. Slowly mix the dry ingredients into the wet ones until they're just combined.
5. Fill each muffin cup about 2/3 full with the batter.
6. Place it in the oven and bake for 18-20 minutes, or until a toothpick inserted in the middle comes out clean.
7. Allow to cool before serving.

Serving Size: 1 muffin

Nutritional Information:

- Calories: 180
- Protein: 4g
- Fat: 8g
- Carbohydrates: 24g
- Fiber: 3g

Pecan Cinnamon Scones

Ingredients:
- 1 cup whole wheat flour
- 1 cup rolled oats
- 1/2 cup pecans, chopped
- 1 teaspoon cinnamon
- 1/2 teaspoon nutmeg
- Pinch of salt
- 1/2 cup butter, softened
- 1/4 cup brown sugar
- 1 large egg

Instructions:
1. Preheat the oven to 375°F (190°C).
2. In a bowl, combine whole wheat flour, rolled oats, chopped pecans, cinnamon, nutmeg, and salt.
3. In a separate bowl, cream together softened butter and brown sugar until light and fluffy.
4. Add the egg to the butter-sugar mixture and mix well.
5. Slowly mix the dry ingredients into the wet ones until they are just combined.
6. Pat the dough into a circle on a floured surface and cut into wedges.
7. Place the wedges on a baking sheet and bake for 15-18 minutes or until the edges are golden.
8. Allow to cool slightly before serving.

Serving Size: 1 scone

Nutritional Information:
- Calories: 220
- Protein: 4g
- Fat: 12g
- Carbohydrates: 25g
- Fiber: 3g

Chocolate Avocado Pudding

Ingredients:
- 2 avocados, ripe
- 1/4 cup cocoa powder
- 1 cup almond milk
- 2 tablespoons honey
- 1 teaspoon vanilla extract

Instructions:
1. In a blender, combine ripe avocados, cocoa powder, almond milk, honey, and vanilla extract.
2. Blend until smooth and creamy.
3. Chill in the refrigerator for a minimum of 2 hours before serving.
4. Spoon into individual serving dishes and garnish with fresh berries or nuts if desired.

Serving Size: 1/2 cup

Nutritional Information:
- Calories: 200
- Protein: 3g
- Fat: 15g
- Carbohydrates: 20g
- Fiber: 7g

Blueberry-Walnut Pancakes

Ingredients:
- 1 cup almond milk
- 1/2 cup frozen blueberries
- 1/4 cup walnuts, chopped
- 1 ripe banana
- 2 tablespoons honey

Instructions:
1. In a blender, combine almond milk, frozen blueberries, chopped walnuts, ripe bananas, and honey.
2. Blend until smooth.
3. Warm up a griddle or non-stick skillet on medium heat.
4. Pour 1/4 cup of batter for each pancake onto the griddle.
5. Cook until bubbles form on the surface, then flip and cook until golden brown on the other side.
6. Repeat with the remaining batter.
7. Serve with an extra drizzle of honey if desired.

Serving Size: 2 pancakes

Nutritional Information:
- Calories: 300
- Protein: 6g
- Fat: 12g
- Carbohydrates: 45g
- Fiber: 6g

Oatmeal Chia Berry Crisp

Ingredients:
- 1 cup oatmeal
- 2 tablespoons chia seeds
- 1 cup frozen berries
- 2 tablespoons honey
- 1 cup almond milk

Instructions:
1. Preheat the oven to 375°F (190°C).
2. In a bowl, combine oatmeal, chia seeds, frozen berries, and honey.
3. Move the mixture into a baking dish.
4. Pour almond milk over the top.
5. Bake for 25-30 minutes or until the top is golden brown.
6. Allow to cool slightly before serving.

Serving Size: 1 cup

Nutritional Information:
- Calories: 250
- Protein: 6g
- Fat: 7g
- Carbohydrates: 40g
- Fiber: 8g

Chapter Eight

Soup and Salad Recipes

Chickpea and Farro Soup with Fennel and Chard

Ingredients:
- 1 cup dried chickpeas, soaked overnight
- 1/2 cup farro
- 1 fennel bulb, diced
- 1 bunch Swiss chard, chopped
- 1 tablespoon olive oil
- Salt and pepper to taste

Instructions:
1. In a big pot, warm olive oil on medium heat.
2. Add diced fennel and sauté until softened.
3. Drain soaked chickpeas and add them to the pot along with farro.
4. Pour in enough water to cover the ingredients and bring to a boil.
5. Reduce heat, cover, and simmer for 45-60 minutes or until chickpeas and farro are tender.
6. Add chopped Swiss chard and cook until wilted.
7. Add salt and pepper to your liking.
8. Serve hot.

Serving Size: 1 cup

Nutritional Information:
- Calories: 200
- Protein: 8g
- Fat: 5g
- Carbohydrates: 32g
- Fiber: 8g

Chicken and Wild Rice Soup

Ingredients:
- 1 cup cooked chicken, shredded
- 1/2 cup wild rice
- 1 carrot, diced
- 1 celery stalk, diced
1-quart chicken broth
- Salt and pepper to taste

Instructions:
1. In a large pot, bring chicken broth to a simmer.
2. Add wild rice and cook until tender.
3. Add shredded chicken, diced carrot, and diced celery.
4. Simmer for an additional 15-20 minutes until vegetables are tender.
5. Season with salt and pepper to taste.
6. Serve hot.

Serving Size: 1 cup
Nutritional Information:
- Calories: 180
- Protein: 15g
- Fat: 4g
- Carbohydrates: 20g
- Fiber: 3g

MIND Diet Minestrone

Ingredients:
- One can (15 oz) of kidney beans, drained and washed
- 1 cup whole wheat pasta, cooked
- 1 cup zucchini, diced
- 1 cup tomatoes, diced
- 1-quart vegetable broth
- 1 teaspoon Italian seasoning

Instructions:
1. In a large pot, combine kidney beans, cooked whole wheat pasta, diced zucchini, and diced tomatoes.
2. Pour in vegetable broth and bring to a simmer.
3. Add Italian seasoning and simmer for 15-20 minutes.
4. Serve hot.

Serving Size: 1 cup

Nutritional Information:
- Calories: 220
- Protein: 10g
- Fat: 2g
- Carbohydrates: 40g
- Fiber: 8g

Tuscan White Bean Soup

Ingredients:
- one can (15 oz) of cannellini beans (drained and washed)
- 1 cup kale, chopped
- 1/2 cup carrots, diced
- 1/2 cup celery, diced
- 1-quart vegetable broth
- 2 tablespoons olive oil

Instructions:
1. In a big pot, warm olive oil on medium heat.
2. Add diced carrots and celery, and sauté until softened.
3. Pour in vegetable broth and add cannellini beans.
4. Bring it to a simmer and let it cook for 15-20 minutes.
5. Add chopped kale and cook until wilted.
6. Serve hot.

Serving Size: 1 cup

Nutritional Information:
- Calories: 180
- Protein: 8g
- Fat: 6g
- Carbohydrates: 25g
- Fiber: 6g

Carrot Soup

Ingredients:
- 1 lb carrots, peeled and chopped
- 1 onion, chopped
- 1-quart vegetable broth
- 1 tablespoon olive oil
- Salt and pepper to taste

Instructions:
1. Warm the olive oil in a big saucepan over medium heat.
2. Saute chopped onions till transparent.
3. Add the chopped carrots and vegetable broth.
4. Bring to a boil, then lower the heat and simmer until the carrots are soft.
5. Puree the soup in an immersion blender until smooth.
6. Season with salt and pepper as desired.

Serving Size: 1 cup

Nutritional Information:
- Calories: 120
- Protein: 2g
- Fat: 4g
- Carbohydrates: 20g
- Fiber: 5g

Black-Eyed Peas Salad

Ingredients:
- One can (15 oz) of black-eyed peas (washed)
- 1 cup cherry tomatoes, halved
- 1/4 cup red onion, finely chopped
- 2 tablespoons olive oil
- 1 tablespoon balsamic vinegar
- Salt and pepper to taste

Instructions:
2. Mix olive oil and balsamic vinegar in a small bowl.
3. Drizzle the dressing over the salad and mix well.
4. Add salt and pepper according to your taste.
5. Serve chilled.

Serving Size: 1 cup

Nutritional Information:
- Calories: 180
- Protein: 8g
- Fat: 7g
- Carbohydrates: 24g
- Fiber: 6g

Kale Kimchi Salad

Ingredients:
- 4 cups kale, chopped
- 1 cup kimchi, chopped
- 1 tablespoon sesame oil
- 1 tablespoon rice vinegar
- 1 teaspoon soy sauce

Instructions:
1. In a large bowl, combine chopped kale and kimchi.
2. In a small bowl, whisk together sesame oil, rice vinegar, and soy sauce.
3. Drizzle the dressing on the salad and mix it well to cover.
4. Massage the kale with the dressing for a few minutes to soften.
5. Serve immediately.

Serving Size: 1 cup

Nutritional Information:
- Calories: 120
- Protein: 5g
- Fat: 6g
- Carbohydrates: 15g
- Fiber: 3g

Cranberry Pear Crisp Salad

Ingredients:
- 4 cups mixed greens
- 1 pear, sliced
- 1/4 cup dried cranberries
- 2 tablespoons chopped walnuts
- 2 tablespoons balsamic vinaigrette dressing

Instructions:
1. In a large bowl, combine mixed greens, sliced pear, dried cranberries, and chopped walnuts.
2. Pour the dressing onto the salad and mix it around to cover everything.
3. Toss to combine.
4. Serve immediately.

Serving Size: 1 cup

Nutritional Information:
- Calories: 180
- Protein: 2g
- Fat: 9g
- Carbohydrates: 25g
- Fiber: 4g

Blueberry Tahini Crisp Salad

Ingredients:
- 4 cups spinach
- 1 cup blueberries
- 2 tablespoons tahini
- 1 tablespoon honey
- 1 tablespoon lemon juice

Instructions:
1. In a large bowl, combine spinach and blueberries.
2. In a small bowl, whisk together tahini, honey, and lemon juice.
3. Pour the dressing onto the salad and mix it thoroughly for an even coating.
4. Serve immediately.

Serving Size: 1 cup

Nutritional Information: (approximate)
- Calories: 160
- Protein: 3g
- Fat: 10g
- Carbohydrates: 18g
- Fiber: 4g

Lovely Lentil Salad with Kale, Cherry Tomatoes, Almonds & Lemon Vinaigrette

Ingredients:
- 1 cup cooked lentils
- 2 cups kale, chopped
- 1 cup cherry tomatoes, halved
- 1/4 cup almonds, chopped
- 2 tablespoons olive oil
- 1 tablespoon lemon juice
- Salt and pepper to taste

Instructions:
1. In a large bowl, combine cooked lentils, chopped kale, cherry tomatoes, and chopped almonds.
2. In a small bowl, whisk together olive oil and lemon juice.
3. Drizzle the dressing on the salad and mix well to cover.
4. Add salt and pepper according to your taste.
5. Serve chilled.

Serving Size: 1 cup

Nutritional Information:
- Calories: 250
- Protein: 13g
- Fat: 12g
- Carbohydrates: 27g
- Fiber: 10g

Chapter Nine

Snacks Recipes

Roasted Chickpeas

Ingredients:
- One can (15 oz) of chickpeas (drained and rinsed)
- 1 tablespoon olive oil
- 1/2 teaspoon salt
- 1/2 teaspoon paprika
- 1/2 teaspoon cumin

Instructions:
1. Preheat the oven to 400°F (200°C).
2. Dry the chickpeas by patting them with a paper towel.
3. In a bowl, toss chickpeas with olive oil, salt, paprika, and cumin.
4. Spread the chickpeas on a baking sheet in a single layer.
5. Roast for 25-30 minutes or until crispy.
6. Allow to cool before serving.

Serving Size: 1/2 cup

Nutritional Information:

- Calories: 120
- Protein: 6g
- Fat: 4g
- Carbohydrates: 16g
- Fiber: 4g

Chocolate Avocado Pudding

Ingredients:
- 2 avocados, ripe
- 1/4 cup cocoa powder
- 1 cup almond milk
- 2 tablespoons honey
- 1 teaspoon vanilla extract

Instructions:
1. In a blender, combine ripe avocados, cocoa powder, almond milk, honey, and vanilla extract.
2. Blend until smooth and creamy.
3. Put it in the fridge for at least 2 hours before you serve it.
4. Spoon into individual serving dishes and garnish with fresh berries or nuts if desired.

Serving Size: 1/2 cup

Nutritional Information:
- Calories: 200
- Protein: 3g
- Fat: 15g
- Carbohydrates: 20g
- Fiber: 7g

Blueberry Almond Smoothie

Ingredients:
- 1 cup blueberries
- 2 tablespoons almond butter
- 1 cup almond milk
- 1 ripe banana
- 1 tablespoon honey

Instructions:
1. Place blueberries, almond butter, almond milk, ripe banana, and honey in a blender.
2. Blend until smooth and nutty.
3. Pour into a glass and enjoy the delightful combination of blueberries and almonds.

Serving Size: 1 cup

Nutritional Information: (approximate)
- Calories: 320
- Protein: 9g
- Fat: 14g
- Carbohydrates: 45g
- Fiber: 8g

Apple Slices with Almond Butter

Ingredients:
- 2 apples, sliced
- 4 tablespoons almond butter

Instructions:
1. Slice the apples into thin wedges.
2. Put almond butter on every slice of the apple.
3. Arrange on a plate and serve.

Serving Size: 1 medium apple with 2 tablespoons almond butter

Nutritional Information:
- Calories: 280
- Protein: 6g
- Fat: 18g
- Carbohydrates: 28g
- Fiber: 7g

Carrot Sticks with Hummus

Ingredients:
- 2 cups carrot sticks
- 1/2 cup hummus

Instructions:
1. Wash and peel carrots, then cut them into sticks.
2. Serve carrot sticks with hummus for dipping.

Serving Size: 1 cup carrot sticks with 1/4 cup hummus

Nutritional Information:
- Calories: 120
- Protein: 4g
- Fat: 7g
- Carbohydrates: 13g
- Fiber: 4g

Trail Mix

Ingredients:
- 1 cup mixed nuts (almonds, walnuts, cashews)
- 1/2 cup mixed of seeds either pumpkin or sunflower seeds)
- 1/2 cup mixed dried fruit (raisins, cranberries, apricots)

Instructions:
1. In a bowl, combine mixed nuts, mixed seeds, and mixed dried fruit.
2. Toss the ingredients until well combined.
3. Portion into small snack-sized bags for easy serving.
4. Enjoy this nutrient-packed trail mix on the go.

Serving Size: 1/4 cup

Nutritional Information: (approximate)
- Calories: 200
- Protein: 6g
- Fat: 12g
- Carbohydrates: 20g
- Fiber: 4g

Greek Yogurt with Berries

Ingredients:
- 1 cup Greek yogurt
- 1/2 cup mixed berries (strawberries, blueberries, raspberries)
- 1 tablespoon honey (optional)

Instructions:
1. Spoon Greek yogurt into a serving bowl.
2. Top with mixed berries.
3. Drizzle honey over the top if desired.
4. Serve chilled.

Serving Size: 1 cup

Nutritional Information:
- Calories: 200
- Protein: 20g
- Fat: 10g
- Carbohydrates: 15g
- Fiber: 2g

8. Roasted Nuts

Ingredients:
- 1 cup mixed nuts (almonds, pecans, cashews)
- 1 tablespoon olive oil
- 1/2 teaspoon salt
- 1/2 teaspoon paprika (optional)

Instructions:
1. Preheat the oven to 350°F (175°C).
2. In a bowl, toss mixed nuts with olive oil, salt, and paprika (if using).
3. Spread the nuts on a baking sheet in a single layer.
4. Roast for 10-12 minutes or until golden brown.
5. Allow to cool before serving.

Serving Size: 1/4 cup

Nutritional Information: (approximate)
- Calories: 200
- Protein: 6g
- Fat: 18g
- Carbohydrates: 6g
- Fiber: 3g

Dark Chocolate

Ingredients:
- 2 ounces dark chocolate (at least 70% cocoa)

Instructions:
1. Break or chop the dark chocolate into bite-sized pieces.
2. Enjoy the dark chocolate as a satisfying and indulgent snack.

Serving Size: 2 ounces

Nutritional Information:
- Calories: 300
- Protein: 4g
- Fat: 20g
- Carbohydrates: 30g
- Fiber: 4g

Popcorn

Ingredients:
- 1/2 cup popcorn kernels
- 1 tablespoon olive oil
- Sprinkle salt

Instructions:
1. In a big pot, warm up olive oil on medium heat.
2. Add popcorn kernels and cover with a lid.
3. Shake the pot occasionally until the popping slows down.
4. Take it off the heat and sprinkle some salt on it.
5. Toss to coat evenly.

Serving Size: 2 cups

Nutritional Information:
- Calories: 100
- Protein: 2g
- Fat: 4g
- Carbohydrates: 15g
- Fiber: 3g

21-Day Meal Plan

Day 1:
- Breakfast: Ultimate Smoothie for Brain Health
- Lunch: Chickpea and Farro Soup with Fennel and Chard
- Snack: Roasted Chickpeas
- Dinner: Cranberry Pear Crisp Salad

Day 2:
- Breakfast: Best Brain Food Smoothie
- Lunch: MIND Diet Minestrone
- Snack: Chocolate Avocado Pudding
- Dinner: Tuscan White Bean Soup

Day 3:
- Breakfast: Blueberry-Walnut Smoothie
- Lunch: Lovely Lentil Salad with Kale, Cherry Tomatoes, Almonds & Lemon Vinaigrette
- Snack: Trail Mix
- Dinner: Carrot Soup

Day 4:
- Breakfast: Chocolate Avocado Pudding
- Lunch: Chicken and Wild Rice Soup
- Snack: Greek Yogurt with Berries
- Dinner: Blueberry Tahini Crisp Salad

Day 5:
- Breakfast: Green Smoothie
- Lunch: Black-Eyed Peas Salad
- Snack: Roasted Nuts
- Dinner: Blueberry Almond Smoothie

Day 6:
- Breakfast: Berry Smoothie
- Lunch: Pecan Cinnamon Scones (Dessert, but can be enjoyed for lunch)
- Snack: Apple Slices with Almond Butter
- Dinner: Pineapple Smoothie

Day 7:
- Breakfast: Whole Grain Blueberry Muffins (Dessert, but can be enjoyed for breakfast)
- Lunch: Blueberry Tahini Crisp Salad
- Snack: Dark Chocolate
- Dinner: Oatmeal Chia Berry Crisp

Day 8:
- Breakfast: Chocolate Avocado Smoothie
- Lunch: Trail Mix
- Snack: Popcorn
- Dinner: Lovely Lentil Salad with Kale, Cherry Tomatoes, Almonds & Lemon Vinaigrette

Day 9:
- Breakfast: Cranberry Pear Crisp Salad
- Lunch: Roasted Nuts
- Snack: Carrot Sticks with Hummus
- Dinner: Chickpea and Farro Soup with Fennel and Chard

Day 10:
- Breakfast: Blueberry Almond Smoothie
- Lunch: MIND Diet Minestrone
- Snack: Greek Yogurt with Berries
- Dinner: Tuscan White Bean Soup

Day 11:
- Breakfast: Best Brain Food Smoothie
- Lunch: Chocolate Avocado Pudding
- Snack: Dark Chocolate
- Dinner: Blueberry Tahini Crisp Salad

Day 12:
- Breakfast: Green Smoothie
- Lunch: Black-Eyed Peas Salad
- Snack: Trail Mix
- Dinner: Blueberry Almond Smoothie

Day 13:
- Breakfast: Berry Smoothie
- Lunch: Pecan Cinnamon Scones (Dessert, but can be enjoyed for lunch)
- Snack: Apple Slices with Almond Butter
- Dinner: Pineapple Smoothie

Day 14:
- Breakfast: Whole Grain Blueberry Muffins (Dessert, but can be enjoyed for breakfast)
- Lunch: Blueberry Tahini Crisp Salad
- Snack: Popcorn
- Dinner: Oatmeal Chia Berry Crisp

Day 15:
- Breakfast: Chocolate Avocado Smoothie
- Lunch: Trail Mix
- Snack: Roasted Nuts
- Dinner: Lovely Lentil Salad with Kale, Cherry Tomatoes, Almonds & Lemon Vinaigrette

Day 16:
- Breakfast: Cranberry Pear Crisp Salad
- Lunch: Roasted Nuts
- Snack: Carrot Sticks with Hummus
- Dinner: Chickpea and Farro Soup with Fennel and Chard

Day 17:
- Breakfast: Blueberry Almond Smoothie
- Lunch: MIND Diet Minestrone
- Snack: Greek Yogurt with Berries
- Dinner: Tuscan White Bean Soup

Day 18:
- Breakfast: Best Brain Food Smoothie
- Lunch: Chocolate Avocado Pudding
- Snack: Dark Chocolate
- Dinner: Blueberry Tahini Crisp Salad

Day 19:
- Breakfast: Green Smoothie
- Lunch: Black-Eyed Peas Salad
- Snack: Trail Mix
- Dinner: Blueberry Almond Smoothie

Day 20:
- Breakfast: Berry Smoothie
- Lunch: Pecan Cinnamon Scones (Dessert, but can be enjoyed for lunch)
- Snack: Apple Slices with Almond Butter
- Dinner: Pineapple Smoothie

Day 21:
- Breakfast: Whole Grain Blueberry Muffins (Dessert, but can be enjoyed for breakfast)
- Lunch: Blueberry Tahini Crisp Salad
- Snack: Popcorn
- Dinner: Oatmeal Chia Berry Crisp

CONCLUSION

As we conclude our culinary adventure through the "MIND Diet Cookbook for Seniors Over 60," I hope you've discovered more than simply a collection of dishes, but a road to feeding both your body and mind. As we appreciate the flavors and embrace the nutritious components, let us also celebrate the delight of living a lifestyle that supports brain health and general well-being. Remember, the MIND diet is more than simply a collection of principles; it is a comprehensive strategy for aging gracefully and with vigor. Each dish in these pages represents a step toward improving cognitive function, including a diverse range of nutrients and enjoying the pleasure of each meal. From vivid smoothies to substantial soups and delicious desserts, the variety of tastes reflects the richness of life at every age.

As we age gracefully, our choices become more important, and the kitchen becomes a sanctuary where we may shape our lifespan. With the MIND diet as our guidance, we can empower ourselves to make conscious decisions not just for our bodies, but also for the inner workings of our brains. So, whether you're enjoying a bowl of Tuscan White Bean Soup or indulging in a guilt-free Chocolate Avocado Pudding, know that you're helping to create a masterpiece of your health.

May this cookbook serve as a guide, motivating you to discover the world of healthy and tasty meals while also connecting the links between nutrition and cognitive vibrancy. As you begin on this tasty adventure, may your kitchen be filled with laughter, your table with shared memories, and your heart with the joy that comes from feeding your body and mind. Let these dishes serve as vivid threads in the big tapestry of life, weaving together a tale of wellness, joy, and age celebration - a gastronomic homage to a life well lived. Cheers to the skill of mindful eating, and to the seniors over 60 who are adopting the MIND diet as a formula for long-term health. Bon appétit, and here's to the lively pages that await!